Leaky Gut Diet:

Low FODMAP Diet - Simple Meal Plans for Leaky Gut and Bowel Disorders

before attempting any techniques outlined in this book.

By reading this document, the reader agrees that under no circumstances are is the author responsible for any losses, direct or indirect, which are incurred as a result of the use of information contained within this document, including, but not limited to, —errors, omissions, or inaccuracies.

Table of Contents

Chapter Three: Snacks

Roasted Chickpeas

Bacon Wrapped Pineapple

Cucumber and Dill Infused Cottage Cheese Appetizer

Sweet Strawberry Treats

Sweet Strawberry Salsa

Buffalo Chicken Meatballs

BBQ Wings

Gorilla Munch Mix Treat

Pineapple Salsa

Grilled Cantaloupe and Prosciutto

Green Bean Bundles

Mediterranean-Style Stuffed Peppers

Maple Pecan Popcorn

Pineapple Walnut Cheese Ball

Roasted Red Peppers, Basil and Fresh Mozzarella

Low FODMAP Antipasto Skewers

Chapter Four: Lunch Recipes

Chapter Five: Dinner Recipes

Chapter Eight: Dips

Conclusion

Introduction

I want to thank you for choosing this book, *'Leaky Gut: Low FODMAP Diet.'*

This recipe book includes a host of new tasty meals for you to enjoy. Some of them are favorites and I have featured them already in my other book, "The Leaky Gut Diet - the Low FODMAP diet made simple."

Over 10% of the world's population suffers from Leaky Gut syndrome. Some of the symptoms of this syndrome include bloating, abdominal pain, diarrhea, constipation or excessive gas. While this disease can be diagnosed easily, it does not necessarily mean that it can be fixed easily. If you are someone who is suffering from these symptoms, this is the perfect book for you.

The Low-FODMAP diet is a diet that has been proven to relieve the symptoms of the syndrome, while also improving the digestion. This program has changed the lives of many people and can work well for you too. FODMAP is an abbreviation that stands for food that is fermentable, short-chain and poorly absorbed carbohydrates. These foods often cause discomfort in the digestive tract. FODMAP stands for Fermentable Oligosaccharides, Disaccharides, Monosaccharides, and Polyols. These terms can overwhelm any reader. All you need to remember is that a saccharide is sugar and oligosaccharides, disaccharides, and monosaccharides are carbohydrates that are made from sugar molecules.

A new diet is always difficult since you will be unaware of the different foods that can be used. You will also need to identify the recipes that adhere to the rules of the diet. This book will help you through your journey. The book contains recipes for every meal of the day. These recipes are simple and easy to make. The first chapter of the book gives you a meal plan for ten days. You can use this plan to test if the diet is indeed for you. Let's get cooking!

I hope you enjoy the recipes in the book.

Chapter One: Meal Plan

We have learned what the low FODMAP diet is and how it will help you control your leaky gut. Now is the time to put everything we have practiced to use and come up with a unique meal plan that will help you control your condition and improve it over time. The recipes mentioned in the meal plan are all elaborately explained and covered in the book. Let us get started!

Day 1

- Breakfast – Zucchini Breakfast Cake
- Lunch – Gluten Free Egg and Cheese Soufflé
- Snack – Sweet and Spicy Barbecue Wings
- Dinner – One Pot Chicken and Rice
- Dessert - Pumpkin Crumb Cake

Day 2

- Breakfast – Pumpkin Spice Smoothie
- Lunch – Spinach, Kale, and Farmer's Cheese Quiche

- Snack – Buffalo Chicken Meatballs
- Dinner – Quiche Lorraine
- Dessert – Frozen banana pops

Day 3

- Breakfast – Blueberry Smoothie Bowl
- Lunch – Peanut Butter and Banana Toast
- Snack – Green Bean Bundles
- Dinner – Mozzarella Chicken
- Dessert - Two Bite Frosted Brownies

Day 4

- Breakfast – Carrot Cake Toast
- Lunch – Mushroom Polenta with Goat's Cheese
- Snack – Pineapple Walnut Cheese Balls
- Dinner – Pork Loin Roast with Herb Stuffing
- Dessert - Chocolate Peanut Butter Bits

Day 5

- Breakfast – Pumpkin Spice Granola Bars
- Lunch – Pork Loin Roast with Herb Stuffing
- Snack – Gorilla Munch Mix Treat

- Dinner – Zucchini Walnut Pancakes and Fruit Salad Smoothie
- Dessert - Creamy Coconut Milk Quinoa Pudding

Day 6

- Breakfast – Blueberry Lime Coconut Smoothie
- Lunch – Chicken Quinoa Meatballs with Soy Sesame Drizzle
- Snack – Maple Pecan Popcorn
- Dinner – Easy One-Pan Ratatouille
- Dessert - Chocolate Chip Cheesecake in a Mug

Day 7

- Breakfast – Gluten Free Waffle Mix
- Lunch – Veggie Cheese Toast with Fresh Spring Rolls
- Snack – Low FODMAP Antipasto Skewers
- Dinner – Mushroom Polenta with Goat's Cheese
- Dessert - Coconut Milk Soft Serve "Ice Cream"

Day 8

- Breakfast – German Pancakes with Berries

- Lunch – Quinoa bowl with Sweet Potato and Tahini Dressing
- Snack – Sweet Strawberry Salsa
- Dinner – Maple and Sesame Chicken with Brown Rice
- Dessert - Double Chocolate Flourless Cookies with Salted Peanuts

Day 9

- Breakfast – Coco-Berry Bowl
- Lunch – Maple and Sesame Chicken with Brown Rice
- Snack – Mediterranean-Style Stuffed Peppers
- Dinner – Pumpkin and Carrot Risotto
- Dessert - Pumpkin Crumb Cake

Day 10

- Breakfast – Chocolate Peanut Butter Smoothie
- Lunch – Carrot and Fennel Soup with Crunchy Roasted Potatoes
- Snack – Sweet Strawberry Treats
- Dinner – Quiche Lorraine with Frosted Brownies
- Dessert - Chocolate Peanut Butter Bits

Chapter Two: Breakfast Recipes

Baked Oatmeal Cups

Serves: 6

Ingredients:

- 1 egg
- ¼ cup water
- 1 teaspoon vanilla extract
- 1 ¼ cups old fashioned oats
- ½ teaspoon ground cinnamon
- 1 tablespoon vegetable oil like canola or grape seed oil
- ½ cup lactose free milk
- 2 ½ tablespoons brown sugar
- 1 teaspoon baking powder

Optional toppings: Use any

- Strawberries, sliced
- Mini semi-sweet chocolate chips
- Almonds or walnuts, chopped
- Cranberries

Method:

1. Place paper liners in a 6-count muffin tin.
2. Add oil, eggs, milk and water into a bowl and whisk well.

3. Add rest of the ingredients and whisk well. Let it rest for 2-3 minutes. Mix again.
4. Divide the batter among the muffin cups. Place the toppings if using.
5. Bake in a preheated oven at 350 °F for 20-25 minutes. It should turn slightly brown on the edges when done.
6. Cool for a while and serve.

Breakfast Cereal Bars

Serves:

Ingredients:

- 2 tablespoons olive oil or coconut oil or butter
- ½ cup natural peanut butter
- 4 cups mini marshmallows without high fructose corn syrup
- 6 cups Mesa Sunrise cereal

Method:

1. Add the fat you are using and marshmallows into a large saucepan. Place saucepan over low heat.
2. Stir constantly until the marshmallows melt.
3. Stir in peanut butter. Stir constantly until smooth. Turn off the heat.
4. Stir in the cereal. Transfer the mixture into a square or rectangular pan. Place a parchment paper on top of the mixture and spread the mixture evenly into the pan, pressing lightly.
5. Refrigerate for 45-60 minutes.
6. Cut into bars and serve.

Breakfast Potatoes

Serves: 4-6

Ingredients:

- 4 large Idaho potatoes, rinsed well
- ½ cup lactose free yogurt
- 4 tablespoons butter, softened
- 2/3 cup sharp cheddar cheese, grated
- 8 bacon strips
- 5-6 slices thin prosciutto
- Salt to taste
- Pepper to taste
- Baby arugula or spinach to top (optional)

Method:

1. Prick the outer surface of the potatoes with a fork at different places.
2. Bake in a preheated oven at 350 °F for 60-75 minutes or until tender.
3. Place the potatoes on your cutting board. Using a kitchen towel, hold the potatoes and cut each into 2 halves. Scoop the flesh of the potatoes and add into a bowl. Place the potatoes on a baking sheet.
4. Add butter, yogurt and cheese into the bowl of scooped potatoes and mash it

until creamy. Fill this mixture into the potato cases.
5. Cook the eggs, bacon and prosciutto in a pan. Top over the potatoes.
6. Bake for 10minutes.
7. Serve hot garnished with baby arugula.

Blueberry Kiwi Minty Groovy Smoothie

Serves: 2

Ingredients:

- 1 cup frozen blueberries
- 2/3 cup lactose free yogurt
- A handful fresh mint leaves (12-15 leaves)
- 2 kiwifruits, peeled, chopped
- 2/3 cup water

Method:

1. Add all the ingredients into a blender and blend until smooth.
2. Pour into tall glasses and serve.

Pineapple Ginger Kale Smoothie

Serves: 2

Ingredients:

- 2 cups nondairy milk of your choice
- 1 ½ cups fresh or frozen pineapple chunks
- 2 inches fresh ginger, peeled, grated or ½ teaspoon dried ginger
- 1 orange, peeled, separated into segments, deseeded
- 2 cups kale
- 2 cups ice

Method:

1. Add all the ingredients into a blender and blend until smooth.
2. Pour into tall glasses and serve.

Potato Scones

Serves: 8

Ingredients:

- 1 ¾ pounds floury potatoes, peeled cubed
- ½ teaspoon salt
- 1 cup self-raising gluten free flour + extra for dusting
- Butter or oil to grease

Method:

1. Place a pot half filled with water over high heat.
2. When it begins to boil, add potatoes and cook until tender.
3. Drain and add potatoes into a bowl. Mash with a potato masher until smooth.
4. Add flour and salt and mix to form dough.
5. Divide the mixture into 6 equal portions.
6. Dust your countertop with some flour. Using a rolling pin, roll into rounds of about ½ cm thick. Cut each into 4 wedges.
7. Place a skillet over medium heat. Add oil or butter. When pan heats, place 3-4 pieces of scones and cook for 3-4

minutes. Flip sides and cook the other side too.

8. Repeat the above step and cook the remaining in batches.
9. Serve with scrambled eggs.

Corn Muffins

Serves: 12

Ingredients:

- 2 cups gluten free all-purpose flour
- 3 tablespoons granulated sugar
- 1 ½ cups lactose free milk
- 3 tablespoons vegetable oil
- 1 cup medium grind corn meal
- 1 teaspoon baking soda
- 3 tablespoons butter, melted, cooled
- 2 eggs, separated

Method:

1. Line a 12-count muffin tin with paper cup liners. Set aside.
2. Add flour, corn meal, baking soda and sugar into a bowl and stir.
3. Stir in milk, yolks, oil and butter and mix until well combined.
4. Beat the whites with a wire whisk until frothy.
5. Pour into the flour mixture. Fold gently.
6. Spoon into muffin molds.
7. Bake in a preheated oven at 375 °F for 18-20 minutes.

Zucchini Breakfast Cake

Serves:

Ingredients:

- 4 cups grated zucchini
- ½ cup oil
- 4 large eggs, whisked
- ½ cup granulated sugar
- 2 teaspoons vanilla extract
- 3 cups gluten free multipurpose flour blend
- 1 teaspoon baking powder
- 1 teaspoon baking soda
- 8 tablespoons melted butter
- 8 ounces lactose free plain yogurt
- 4 tablespoons brown sugar
- 2/3 cup coconut, unsweetened (optional)
- 1 teaspoon almond extract
- 2/3 cup almonds, sliced

For glaze:

- 1 cup confectioner's sugar
- Water, as required
- ½ teaspoon almond extract

Method:

1. Grease a baking dish with oil or butter.

2. Add eggs into a bowl and whisk well. Add zucchini, butter, yogurt and oil and whisk until well combined.
3. Add sugars, coconut, almond extract and vanilla extract and whisk well.
4. Add flour, baking powder and baking soda and mix well.
5. Add almonds and fold gently. Spoon into the prepared baking dish.
6. Bake in a preheated oven at 375 °F for 20 minutes or a toothpick, when inserted in the center, comes out clean.
7. Meanwhile, make the glaze as follows: Add all the ingredients of glaze into a bowl and whisk well. Add a couple of teaspoons of water if required. Pour over the cake.
8. Slice and serve.

Pumpkin Spice Granola Bars

Makes: 5 bars

Ingredients:

- 1 cup oats
- ¼ cup walnuts, chopped
- 3 tablespoons maple syrup
- 2 tablespoons shredded coconut
- ½ teaspoon ground allspice
- 2 tablespoons brown sugar
- ¼ cup canned pumpkin
- ½ tablespoon coconut oil
- ½ teaspoon ground cinnamon

Method:

1. Grease a small square pan with oil or butter.
2. Add all the ingredients into a bowl and whisk well.
3. Spoon into the prepared pan.
4. Bake in a preheated oven at 375 °F for 20-30 minutes.
5. Cool completely. Slice into 5 equal bars. Chill for an hour or two.

Carrot Cake Toast

Serves: 4

Ingredients:

- 1 cup shredded carrots
- 1 tablespoon cinnamon sugar
- Chopped walnuts to garnish
- ¼ teaspoon vanilla extract
- ¼ cup lactose free cream cheese
- 4 slices gluten free bread, toasted

Method:

1. Place bread slices on a serving platter.
2. Add rest of the ingredients into a bowl and mix well.
3. Spread over the toasts and serve right away.

Ham and Egg Toast

Serves: 4

Ingredients:

- 4 eggs, hard boiled, sliced
- 2 teaspoons Dijon mustard
- Peppered ham slices
- 4 teaspoons butter
- 4 tablespoons cheddar cheese, shredded
- 4 slices gluten free bread, toasted

Method:

1. Spread 1-teaspoon butter on each bread slice. Spread ½ teaspoon Dijon mustard over it.
2. Place ham slices and finally sprinkle cheddar cheese on top and serve.

German Pancake with Berries

Serves:

Ingredients:

- ½ cup gluten free flour blend
- ½ cup oat flour
- 6 large eggs, whisked
- 2 tablespoons sugar
- 1 cup lactose free milk
- ½ teaspoon vanilla or almond extract (optional)

<u>Toppings:</u> Use any, as required

- Strawberries, sliced
- Butter, melted
- Blueberries
- Confectioner's sugar

Method:

1. Grease a cast iron skillet with a little oil or butter.
2. Add flours, milk, eggs, sugar and the extract you are using into a bowl. Whisk until well combined and smooth.
3. Spoon into the skillet.
4. Bake in a preheated oven at 450 °F for 12 minutes or until the pancake puffs. Cut into wedges.
5. Place toppings you are using and serve.

Gluten Free Waffle Mix

Makes: 7 cups

Ingredients:

<u>For waffle mix:</u>

- 6 cups gluten free flour blend
- 3 teaspoons baking powder
- 1 teaspoon salt
- 2/3 cup sugar
- 2 teaspoons baking soda

<u>Serving day:</u>

- 2 cups waffle mix
- 3 tablespoons vegetable oil or melted butter + extra to grease
- 2 eggs
- 1 1/3 cups lactose free milk

Method:

1. Add all the ingredients of waffle mix in an airtight container. Mix well. Close the lid. Store in a cool and dry place.
2. On serving day: Add 2 cups waffle mix, eggs, lactose free milk and vegetable oil into a bowl and whisk well. Let it sit for 10 minutes. Whisk again.
3. Place a nonstick griddle or pan over medium heat. Add a little butter and grease the pan.

4. Pour about ¼ cup of batter on the pan. Swirl the pan so that the batter spreads. Bubbles will form on the top. Cook until the underside is golden brown, flip sides and cook the other side too.
5. Repeat the above 2 steps with the remaining batter.
6. Serve with toppings of your choice.

*** While making fruit based smoothies, use lesser fruits than mentioned in the recipes if you cannot tolerate the fruits or replace with fruits that suit you***

Pumpkin Spice Smoothie

Serves: 2

Ingredients:

- ½ cup canned pumpkin
- ½ teaspoon ginger, peeled, grated
- 1 teaspoon allspice
- 4 teaspoons pure maple syrup
- Ice cubes, as required
- ½ cup canned light coconut milk or almond milk
- ½ teaspoon ground cinnamon
- 2 teaspoons vanilla
- 4 tablespoons plain Greek yogurt or lactose free yogurt, as per your tolerance
- Pure maple syrup or cinnamon sugar to garnish

Method:

1. Place all the ingredients into a blender and blend until smooth.
2. Pour into tall glasses and serve.

Blueberry Lime Coconut Smoothie

Serves: 2

Ingredients:

- 1 cup blueberries, fresh or frozen
- 4 tablespoons fresh lime juice
- 2 teaspoons chia seeds
- Ice, to be used if using fresh blueberries
- 4 tablespoons flaked coconut
- 8 ounces plain nonfat lactose free yogurt
- ¼ cup water

Method:

1. Place all the ingredients into a blender and blend until smooth.
2. Pour into tall glasses and serve.

Fruit Salad Smoothie

Serves: 2

Ingredients:

- 2 cups frozen mixed fruits of your choice
- ¼ cup light coconut milk
- ¼ teaspoon lemon zest, grated (optional)
- A handful walnuts, finely chopped, to top
- ¼ cup lemon Chobani yogurt or any lactose free yogurt
- Water, as required, to dilute
- 4 teaspoons shredded coconut, to top

Method:

1. Set aside the toppings and add rest of the ingredients into a blender and blend until smooth.
2. Pour into tall glasses. Sprinkle coconut and walnuts on top and serve.

Chocolate Peanut Butter Smoothie

Serves: 2

Ingredients:

- 2 bananas, peeled, sliced, frozen
- 2 tablespoons oats
- 2 teaspoons ground cinnamon
- 4 teaspoons cocoa powder
- 1 cup lactose free milk or almond milk

Method:

1. Place all the ingredients in a blender and blend until smooth.
2. Pour into tall glasses and serve.

Blueberry Kale Smoothie

Serves: 2

Ingredients:

- 12 ounces Greek yogurt or lactose free yogurt
- 2 teaspoons pure maple syrup
- 1 cup kale leaves, discard hard ribs and stems, torn
- 2 tablespoons lemon juice
- Ice cubes, as required
- 4 tablespoons canned light coconut milk
- 40 frozen blueberries
- 2 tablespoons pumpkin seeds
- 2 tablespoons water

Method:

1. Place all the ingredients in a blender and blend until smooth.
2. Pour into tall glasses and serve.

Blueberry Smoothie Bowl

Serves: 2

Ingredients:

<u>For smoothie:</u>

- 20 blueberries
- 2 teaspoons chia seeds
- Ice cubes
- 8 ounces plain yogurt or lactose free yogurt
- ½ cup lactose free milk
- Ice cubes, as required

<u>For topping:</u>

- 8 thin slices banana
- 4 teaspoons chia seeds
- Blueberries, as required
- 2 tablespoons hulled pumpkin seeds (pepitas)

Method:

1. Add all the ingredients of smoothie into a blender and blend until smooth.
2. Pour into 2 serving bowls.
3. Place the toppings in rows on the smoothie bowls and serve.

Coco-Berry Bowl

Serves: 2

Ingredients:

- 6 strawberries, frozen
- 20 blueberries, frozen
- 2 tablespoons chia seeds + extra to garnish
- ¼ cup canned, light coconut milk
- 2 teaspoons shredded coconut, to garnish

Method:

1. Add berries, chia seeds, yogurt and coconut milk into a blender and blend until smooth.
2. Pour into 2 bowls. Sprinkle chia seeds and shredded coconut and serve.

Chapter Three: Snacks

Carrot and Parsnip Chips

Serves:

Ingredients:

- 2 large or medium carrots, peeled, trimmed
- 2 large or 4 medium parsnips, peeled, trimmed
- Olive oil cooking spray
- 2 teaspoons thyme leaves, chopped (optional)
- Salt to taste

Method:

1. Make long strips of the carrots and parsnips using a 'Y' shaped vegetable peeler.
2. Spread it on a greased baking sheet. Spray with cooking spray.
3. Sprinkle salt and thyme leaves.
4. Bake in a preheated oven at 325 °F for 35 minutes. Turn the chips a couple of times while baking.

Bacon Wrapped Pineapple

Serves: 10

Ingredients:

- 5 slices precooked bacon, halved
- ½ tablespoon pure maple syrup
- 10 bite size pieces pineapple

Method:

1. Place bacon slices in the microwave and microwave on high for 15 seconds.
2. Place bacon slices on a baking sheet. Place a piece of pineapple on each slice of bacon at one end. Wrap and fasten with a toothpick. Drizzle maple syrup over it.
3. Bake in a preheated oven at 350 °F for 5-10 minutes.

Roasted Chickpeas

Serves: 8 (¼ cup each)

Ingredients:

- 2 cans chickpeas, drained, rinsed
- ½ teaspoon freshly ground pepper
- ½ teaspoon salt
- 1 teaspoon dried rosemary, crushed
- ½ teaspoon smoked sweet paprika
- 2 teaspoons olive oil
- 1 teaspoon garlic powder
- ½ teaspoon dried thyme

Method:

1. Dry the chickpeas with a clean kitchen towel.
2. Add chickpeas into a bowl. Drizzle oil over it and toss well.
3. Sprinkle seasonings on top and toss until well coated.
4. Line a baking sheet with aluminum foil. Spread the chickpeas on it in a single layer.
5. Bake in a preheated oven at 450° F for about 30-45 minutes. Toss 2-3 times while it is baking. Bake until it is turning light brown in color.
6. Remove the baking sheet from the oven after 15-20 minutes.

7. Cool completely. Transfer into an airtight container and store until use.

Cucumber and Dill-infused Cottage Cheese Appetizer

Serves:

Ingredients:

- 2 large cucumbers, trimmed, cut into 1 ½ inch thick round slices
- 4 teaspoons garlic infused oil
- 2 scallions, thinly slice the green parts only, to garnish
- 1 ½ cups lactose free cottage cheese
- 4 teaspoons fresh dill, chopped or 1 teaspoon dried dill
- Coarsely ground pepper to taste

Method:

1. Place the cucumber rounds on a serving platter. Carefully scoop out some of the seeds and flesh from the cucumber rounds, keeping the base intact.
2. Mix together in a bowl, cottage cheese, dill and garlic infused oil. Divide the mixture and fill in the cucumber cases.
3. Sprinkle scallions and pepper powder and serve.

Sweet Strawberry Treats

Serves:

Ingredients:

- 2 quarts strawberries, rinsed but do not hull
- ½ cup brown sugar or maple sugar
- ½ cup Greek yogurt or lactose free sour cream or plain lactose free yogurt

Method:

1. First, dip strawberries in sour cream and then dredge in brown sugar or maple sugar.
2. Serve right away.

Sweet Strawberry Salsa

Serves:

Ingredients:

- 3 cups strawberries, hulled, chopped
- 4 teaspoons balsamic vinegar
- 2 green onions, green parts cut into thin slices
- 2 cup grape tomatoes, quartered
- 2 tablespoons olive oil
- A handful fresh cilantro, chopped

Method:

1. Add strawberries, vinegar, green onions, tomatoes and oil into a bowl and toss well.
2. Sprinkle cilantro on top and serve with corn tortilla chips.

Buffalo Chicken Meatballs

Serves: 8-10

Ingredients:

- 2 pounds ground chicken breast
- 4 tablespoons butter
- 1 1/3 cups Glutino plain bread crumbs or its alternative
- 2 eggs

Method:

1. Place chicken in a bowl.
2. Add butter into a saucepan. Place saucepan over medium heat. When it melts, turn off the heat and add hot sauce.
3. Pour over the chicken. Add breadcrumbs, celery and eggs. Mix well.
4. Make balls of the mixture of about 1 ½ inches diameter. Place on a greased baking sheet.
5. Bake in a preheated oven at 375 °F for 25-30 minutes or until done. Turn the balls half way through baking.
6. Insert toothpicks and serve.

BBQ Wings

Serves: 4

Ingredients:

- 8 chicken wings, trimmed, cut for wing appetizers
- 1 tablespoon Casa de Sante BBQ rub
- 1 teaspoon olive oil

Method:

1. Place wings on a baking sheet. Brush with oil. Rub ½ tablespoon BBQ rub all over the wings.
2. Bake in a preheated oven at 375 °F for 25-30 minutes.
3. Flip sides and sprinkle remaining rub over it.
4. Bake for another 5-6 minutes.

Gorilla Munch Mix Treat

Makes: ½ cup servings

Ingredients:

- ¾ cup semi-sweet chocolate chips
- 3 cups gluten free pretzels
- 1 ½ cups salted peanuts
- 3 cups Gorilla Munch (Nature's path)
- 1/3 cup pepitas (pumpkin seeds)

Method:

1. Add all the ingredients into an airtight container. Close the lid and shake the container to mix well.
2. Serve.

Pineapple Salsa

Serves: 3-4

Ingredients:

<u>For salsa:</u>

- ½ cup fresh pineapple, diced
- 2 tablespoons chopped green bell pepper
- ½ teaspoon lime zest
- ½ tablespoon lime juice
- ½ tablespoon parsley or cilantro, chopped
- ¼ cup cherry tomatoes, quartered
- 1 small jalapeño, deseeded, diced
- ½ tablespoon olive oil
- Salt to taste
- Pepper to taste

<u>To serve:</u>

- Corn tortillas, freshly grilled
- Chicken or beef strips or grilled shrimp
- Grated cheddar cheese

Method:

1. Add all the ingredients of salsa into a bowl. Toss well. Cover and chill overnight.

2. Freshly grill corn tortillas. Spread salsa over the tortillas.
3. Place chicken or beef strips or grilled shrimp over it. Sprinkle cheese on top and serve.

Grilled Cantaloupe and Prosciutto

Serves: 4

Ingredients:

- 8 slices cantaloupe
- 8 thin slices prosciutto
- Toothpicks soaked in water

Method:

1. Wrap a prosciutto slice over each cantaloupe slice. Fasten with toothpicks and serve.

Green Bean Bundles

Serves: 8

Ingredients:

- 80-100 green beans, trimmed
- ½ pound provolone cheese, thinly sliced into 1 inch strips
- 2 tablespoons parmesan cheese, grated
- ½ pound thinly sliced imported ham, cut into 1 inch strips
- 2 tablespoons garlic infused oil

Method:

1. Gather similarly sized beans together.
2. To make 1 set, take 3 green beans. Wrap ham and cheese in the center and place on a lined baking sheet.
3. Similarly, make the remaining sets.
4. Brush with garlic infused oil.
5. Bake in a preheated oven at 375 °F for 25-30 minutes or until tender.
6. Sprinkle Parmesan cheese and serve.

Mediterranean-Style Stuffed Peppers

Serves: 6

Ingredients:

- 8 medium bell peppers or any color or mixed colors or use more of mini bell peppers
- 4 tablespoons olive oil
- 4 tablespoons soy sauce
- ½ cup fresh mint, chopped
- 1 ½ cups feta cheese, crumbled
- 3 cups brown rice couscous or brown rice, cooked
- 2 pounds ground turkey breast
- 8 scallions, green parts only
- 4 tablespoons fresh lemon juice

Method:

1. Place a large skillet over medium heat. Add oil. When the oil is heated, add turkey and cook until done.
2. Add couscous or brown rice and stir.
3. Add soy sauce, mint leaves, scallions, feta and lemon juice. And fold gently.
4. Turn off the heat. Fill the peppers with the mixture. Place the peppers in a baking dish, with the filled side facing down.
5. Cover the dish with foil.

6. Bake in a preheated oven at 350 °F for 25-30 minutes or until tender.

Maple Pecan Popcorn

Serves: 3

Ingredients:

- 3 cups popped popcorn
- ½ cup pecans
- 6 tablespoons firmly packed brown sugar
- 1/8 teaspoon baking soda
- ¼ cup pepitas, toasted
- 3 tablespoons butter
- 1 tablespoon maple syrup
- ½ teaspoon vanilla extract

Method:

1. Line a baking sheet with parchment paper. Spread popcorn over the baking sheet. Also, spread the nuts or seeds.
2. Add butter, maple syrup and sugar into a saucepan. Place the saucepan over medium heat. Stir frequently until it melts.
3. Lower heat and simmer for 5 minutes. Turn off the heat.
4. Add vanilla and baking soda and stir. Drizzle over the popcorn. Let it cool for a while.
5. Serve.

Pineapple Walnut Cheese Ball

Serves: 16-20

Ingredients:

- 1 tin crushed pineapple, drained
- 4 tablespoons green onions, green part only, sliced
- 2 containers (8 ounces each) Green Valley lactose free cream cheese, at room temperature
- 2 cups walnuts, chopped

Method:

1. Line a tray with parchment paper.
2. Add pineapple and cream cheese into a bowl and mix well.
3. Add green onions and fold gently.
4. Divide the mixture into 16-20 equal portions and shape into balls.
5. Place walnuts on a plate. Dredge the rolls in walnuts and place on the prepared baking sheet.
6. Cover the baking sheet with cling wrap and refrigerate until use.
7. Serve over crackers if desired or with a dip of your choice.

Roasted Red Peppers, Basil and Fresh Mozzarella

Serves: 6

Ingredients:

- 2 roasted red peppers, chopped into small strips
- ½ cup fresh basil, to garnish
- 3-4 teaspoons red wine vinegar
- Salt to taste
- Pepper to taste
- 12 mini mozzarella balls
- 2 tablespoons olive oil

Method:

1. Add all the ingredients in a bowl and toss well.
2. Serve 2 balls per serving.

Low FODMAP Antipasto Skewers

Serves:

Ingredients:

- 2 small jars pepperoncini
- 2 small containers fresh small mozzarella balls
- ½ cup fresh basil leaves, rinsed, slice each leaf into 2 halves
- Small bamboo skewers, of about 6 inches length
- 2 small jars kalamata olives, pitted
- Thinly sliced prosciutto, cut in thirds lengthwise
- 2 small containers grape tomatoes

Method:

1. If there are large size pepperoncini's, cut into 2 halves.
2. Fold prosciutto in such a manner that it is a square. Insert the skewer through it.
3. Insert all the remaining ingredients in any manner you desire onto the skewers.
4. Place on a serving platter and serve.

Chapter Four: Lunch Recipes

Potato Salad with Anchovy and Quail's Eggs

Serves: 2

Ingredients:

- 8 quail's eggs
- 7 ounces new potatoes, halved or quartered, depending on the size
- 7 ounces green beans
- A handful fresh parsley, chopped
- Juice of a lemon
- 2 anchovies, finely chopped
- 2 tablespoons chopped chives

Method:

1. Place a pot over medium heat. Pour enough water to fill up to about ¾.
2. When it begins to boil, gently lower the eggs into the water. Let it simmer for 2 minutes and 15 seconds for soft boiled.
3. Remove the eggs with a slotted spoon and plunge in a bowl of cold water.
4. Add beans into the simmering water in the pot and cook for 4 minutes. Remove

beans and submerge in a bowl of cold water.

5. Now add potatoes to the simmering water. Cook until tender. Discard the water and place potatoes in a colander. Let it cool.
6. Peel and halve the eggs.
7. Add potatoes, beans, anchovies, lemon juice, parsley and chives into a bowl and toss well.
8. Divide into individual plates. Place eggs on top and serve.

Low FODMAP Chicken Noodle Soup

Serves: 6-8

Ingredients:

- 4-6 cups low FODMAP chicken broth
- 2 cups chopped, cooked chicken breast
- Salt to taste
- Pepper to taste
- 4-6 cups water
- 4-8 ounces raw gluten free pasta / noodles like brown rice pasta fusilli

Method:

1. Pour broth and water into a pot. Place the pot over medium heat. Stir frequently.
2. When it begins to boil, add pasta, salt, pepper and chicken and cook until pasta is al dente.
3. Ladle into soup bowls and serve.

Egg Wraps

Serves: 2

Ingredients:

- 4 egg whites
- 2 eggs
- Pepper to taste
- Salt to taste
- Toppings of your choice that are low FODMAP friendly

Method:

1. Whisk together in a bowl, whites, eggs, salt and pepper.
2. Place a nonstick pan over medium heat. Spray with cooking spray. Pour half the egg mixture.
3. Cook for 2-3 minutes. Flip sides and cook the other side too.
4. Carefully slide on to a plate. Place toppings of your choice and wrap. Serve right away.
5. Repeat the above 3 steps to make the other wrap.

Poached Egg Sandwich with Smoked Salmon

Serves: 2

Ingredients:

- 4 fresh eggs
- ¼ avocado
- Lemon juice to taste
- Rocket lettuce (optional)
- 3.5 ounces smoked salmon
- Pepper to taste
- Salt to taste
- 4 slices sourdough spelt bread

Method:

1. Add avocado, lemon juice, salt and pepper into a bowl and mash well with a fork.
2. Smear this on one side of the bread slices.
3. Place salmon on each of the slices. Place rocket leaves on top.
4. Place a pan of water over high heat. When the water begins to boil, lower heat. Crack the eggs in it and poach the eggs. Remove carefully and place over the sandwiches. Season with salt and pepper and serve.

Buckwheat Pancakes

Makes: 5-6

Ingredients:

- 3.5 ounces buckwheat flour
- A small pinch salt
- 10 ounces lactose free milk
- 1 egg, at room temperature
- Cooking spray
- Toppings of your choice that are low FODMOP friendly

Method:

1. Add buckwheat flour and salt into a bowl. Add egg and whisk until well combined.
2. Add milk, a little at a time and whisk well.
3. Place a nonstick pan or griddle over medium heat. Spray with cooking spray,
4. Pour about ¼ cup batter over it. Swirl the pan so that the batter spreads. Cook until the underside is golden brown. Flip sides and cook the other side too.
5. Place toppings of your choice and serve.

Veggie and Cheese Toast

Serves: 4

Ingredients:

- ½ cup lactose free cottage cheese
- ½ teaspoon lemon zest, grated
- ¼ cup red bell pepper, chopped
- Pepper to taste
- Red pepper flakes to taste
- 4 slices gluten free bread, toasted

Method:

1. Place bread slices on a serving platter.
2. Add rest of the ingredients into a bowl and mix well.
3. Spread over the toasts and serve right away.

Peanut Butter and Banana Toast

Serves: 4

Ingredients:

- 1 banana, peeled, thinly sliced
- 4 tablespoons peanut butter
- 4 teaspoons chia seeds
- Pepita (hulled pumpkin seeds) to garnish
- 4 slices gluten free bread, toasted
- Maple syrup to drizzle

Method:

1. Spread a tablespoon of peanut butter on each slice of bread.
2. Place banana slices over it. Sprinkle chia seeds and pepita and serve drizzled with maple syrup.

Gluten Free Egg and Cheese Soufflé

Serves:

Ingredients:

- 10 slices gluten free bread
- 8 eggs
- 2 cups cheddar cheese or Pepper Jack cheese
- 3 teaspoons yellow mustard
- 4 tablespoons butter
- 4 cups milk
- 3 teaspoons gluten free Worcestershire sauce
- 2 tablespoons fresh chives, finely chopped

Method:

1. Spread butter over the bread slices and then cut each slice into 6 cubes.
2. Place in a casserole dish.
3. Add eggs, Worcestershire sauce, milk and mustard in a bowl and whisk well.
4. Pour over the bread cubes. Cover the dish with cling wrap. Place dish in the refrigerator for 6-8 hours.
5. Remove from the refrigerator an hour before baking.
6. Bake in a preheated oven at 375 °F for 40-50 minutes or until brown on top.

Zucchini Walnut Pancakes

Serves: 4-6

Ingredients:

- 2 cups gluten free pancake mixture
- 1 cup lactose free milk
- 2 cups zucchini, grated
- ½ teaspoon ground cinnamon
- 2 eggs
- 2 teaspoons sugar
- 2 teaspoons vanilla extract
- ½ cups walnuts, chopped

Method:

1. Add all the ingredients into a blender and blend until smooth.
2. Place a nonstick griddle over medium heat. Grease with a little oil.
3. Make 2-3 small pancakes over it. Cook until the underside is golden brown.
4. Flip sides and cook the other side too.
5. Repeat the above 3 steps with the remaining batter.

Spinach, Kale & Farmer's Cheese Quiche

Serves: 8-9

Ingredients:

- 1 large gluten free pie crust
- 1 ½ cups fresh baby spinach or kale, chopped
- 9 extra-large eggs, beaten
- 3 spring onions, green parts only, chopped
- 1 ½ cups farmer's cheese
- 1 ½ teaspoons thyme
- ¾ cup lactose free milk
- Salt to taste

Method:

1. Spread farmer's cheese on the piecrust.
2. Mix together spinach, kale and thyme in a bowl and sprinkle over the piecrust.
3. Whisk together eggs and milk in a bowl and pour over the spinach and kale.
4. Scatter greens of scallion on top. Place on a baking sheet.
5. Bake in a preheated oven at 350 °F for 40-50 minutes or until brown on top.

Chicken Quinoa Meatballs with Soy Sesame Drizzle

Serves: 10-15

Ingredients:

<u>For meatballs:</u>

- 2 pounds ground chicken breast
- 2 egg yolks
- 2 tablespoons sesame oil
- 2 tablespoons hot sauce
- ½ cup soy sauce
- 2 tablespoons fresh ginger, grated
- 4 cups cooked quinoa

<u>For soy sesame drizzle:</u>

- ½ cup soy sauce
- 2 tablespoons fresh ginger, freshly grated
- 2 teaspoons sesame oil
- 2 tablespoons rice wine vinegar
- 2 tablespoons light brown sugar
- 2 teaspoons cornstarch mixed with ½ cup water

<u>To garnish:</u>

- ½ cup fresh cilantro, chopped
- 2 scallions, green parts only, chopped
- 2 tablespoons sesame seeds

Method:

1. Grease a large baking sheet with a little oil.
2. Add all the meatball ingredients into a bowl and mix well. Shape into meatballs.
3. Place on a baking sheet. Use more baking sheets if required and bake in batches.
4. Bake in a preheated oven at 350 °F for 18-20 minutes or until brown and cooked. Turn the meatballs half way through baking.
5. Meanwhile, make the soy sesame drizzle as follows:
6. Add all the ingredients of soy sesame drizzle except cornstarch mixture into a saucepan.
7. Place the saucepan over medium heat. When the mixture is heated, add cornstarch mixture stirring constantly. Stir until thick. Turn off the heat.
8. Place the cooked meatballs in a large bowl. Drizzle the soy sesame drizzle over the meatballs.
9. Garnish with cilantro, scallions and sesame seeds and serve.

Asian Salad and Sesame Chicken Spring Roll

Serves: 20

Ingredients:

- 2 chicken breasts, skinless, boneless, cut each into 10 even strips
- 6 teaspoons sesame oil
- 4 teaspoons sesame seeds
- 4 medium carrots, peeled, trimmed, cut into matchsticks
- 2 medium summer squash, trimmed, peeled, cut into matchsticks
- 1 English cucumber, peeled, trimmed, cut into matchsticks
- 1/3 cup fresh cilantro, chopped
- 6 ounces rice sticks (noodles)
- 5 tablespoons low sodium soy sauce
- 2 teaspoons fresh ginger, minced
- 2 tablespoons peanut oil
- 4 teaspoons rice wine vinegar
- 20 spring roll wrappers

Method:

1. Place chicken strips in a glass bowl. Add 2 tablespoons soy sauce, 2 teaspoons sesame oil, sesame seeds and ginger. Toss well. Cover and set aside for 15-20 minutes.

2. You can also cut the vegetables using a julienne peeler.
3. Place a skillet over medium heat. Add oil. When the oil is heated, add only the chicken (without marinade).
4. Cook until tender.
5. Add ¼ cup cilantro, 2 teaspoons rice wine vinegar, 1 teaspoon sesame oil and 2 teaspoons soy sauce into a bowl. Add carrots into it.
6. Cook the noodles following the directions on the package. Sprinkle 4 teaspoons sesame oil over it.
7. Add very warm water into a large bowl. Hydrate one spring roll wrapper at a time until malleable.
8. Place the wrappers on your countertop. Place some chicken, vegetables and noodles on one of the longer edges. Roll the spring roll like the way you roll a burrito.
9. Add all of the remaining- soy sauce, sesame oil, cilantro and vinegar into a bowl and stir. Use this as a dip.
10. Place spring rolls on your cutting board and cut them into pieces, diagonally.

Hash Browns with Gruyere and Pancetta

Serves:

Ingredients:

- ¾ pound Maris Piper or King Edward potatoes, peeled, chopped into chunks
- 2 teaspoons chopped chives
- 2 tablespoons Gruyere cheese, grated
- 1 large egg, lightly beaten
- 2 teaspoons olive oil
- 1.5 ounces pancetta, diced
- A handful fresh parsley, chopped
- Salt to taste
- Freshly ground pepper to taste

Method:

1. Place a saucepan half filled with water over medium heat. Add a little salt. When it begins to boil, add potatoes and cook until tender. Drain and add it back into the saucepan. Place the saucepan over medium heat. Turn off the heat when all the moisture dries up. Let it cool for a while.
2. Meanwhile, place a skillet over medium heat. Add 1-teaspoon oil. When the oil is

heated, add pancetta and cook until crisp.

3. Chop the potatoes into 1 cm cubes and add into a bowl. Add rest of the ingredients and stir.
4. Place a nonstick pan over medium heat. Add the potato mixture on the pan. Press with the back of a spoon.
5. Cook until the underside is golden brown. Flip sides and cook the other side too.
6. Serve with roasted tomatoes.

Chapter Five: Dinner Recipes

Sweet and Sour Chicken

Serves: 8

Ingredients:

- 2 pounds chicken breasts, skinless, boneless, cut into 1 inch pieces
- 2 large eggs, beaten
- 1 cup coconut sugar or regular white sugar
- 4 tablespoons coconut aminos or tamari
- ½ cup chicken stock
- 2 cups pineapple chunks
- 1 cup arrowroot starch or cornstarch
- ½ cup coconut oil
- ½ cup apple cider vinegar or white wine or rice vinegar
- ½ cup ketchup or Low FODMAP ketchup
- 2 red peppers, cut into 1 inch squares
- 6 spring onions, green parts only, thinly sliced
- Oil, as required

Method:

1. To make sauce: Add coconut sugar, coconut aminos, vinegar, stock and

ketchup into a saucepan. Place the saucepan over medium heat. Stir frequently.

2. When it begins to boil, lower heat and let it simmer.
3. Add chicken into the bowl of eggs. Stir until well coated. Sprinkle some arrowroot over it. Toss and sprinkle again. Toss until the pieces are well coated.
4. Place a large skillet over medium heat. Add oil. When the oil is heated, add chicken and cook until slightly crisp on all the sides.
5. Add red pepper and pineapple and stir. Cook until chicken is brown and tender from inside.
6. Pour the simmering sauce over the chicken. Stir and lower heat.
7. Cover and simmer for 3-5 minutes. Turn off heat.
8. Add green onions and stir. Serve with rice.

Baked Lemon Pepper Chicken & Rice

Serves: 6

Ingredients:

- 6 chicken breasts, skinless, boneless, thinly sliced
- 6 tablespoons butter or vegan butter, melted
- 1 ½ cups basmati rice
- 2 tablespoons lemon pepper seasoning or to taste
- 28 ounces chicken broth
- 1 teaspoon salt (do not add if the chicken broth is salted)

Method:

1. Sprinkle lemon pepper seasoning all over the chicken.
2. Add butter into a large baking dish. Swirl the dish so that butter spreads all over.
3. Place chicken in the dish. Cover the dish with foil.
4. Bake in a preheated oven at 350° F for about 30-45 minutes or until tender. Flip sides after about 15-18 minutes during baking.

5. Remove chicken from the dish and place on a plate. Cover the plate and keep it warm.
6. Add broth, rice and salt into the same dish. Cover the dish with foil.
7. Bake for 30 minutes or until rice is cooked. Place chicken on top. Cover with foil.
8. Bake for another 15-20 minutes.
9. Serve hot.

Beef Skillet Supper

Serves: 6

Ingredients:

- 2 pounds grass fed ground beef
- 1 medium cabbage, sliced (optional)
- 2 teaspoons fresh ginger, peeled, grated
- 2 medium zucchinis, very thinly sliced, preferably with a mandolin slicer
- 2 scallions, green parts only, thinly sliced, to garnish
- 3 cups white sweet potato, diced
- 2 large carrots, very thinly sliced, preferably with a mandolin slicer
- A handful fresh cilantro or parsley, chopped to garnish
- 2 teaspoons duck fat or bacon fat or lard or more if required
- 6 tablespoons coconut aminos
- Sea salt to taste

Method:

1. Place a large skillet over medium high heat (preferably cast iron skillet). Add fat.
2. When fat melts, add beef and cook until light brown.

3. Stir in coconut aminos, ginger, sweet potato and cabbage.
4. Cover and cook until sweet potatoes are tender. Stir occasionally. Remove from heat.
5. Add carrots and zucchini and stir until well combined. Cover and let it sit for a few minutes.
6. Place the skillet back on heat for a couple of minutes if you like the carrots and zucchini more cooked.
7. Divide into plates. Sprinkle scallion, cilantro and salt and serve.

Sardine Spaghetti with Tomato- Caper Sauce

Serves: 6

Ingredients:

- 4 tablespoons extra- virgin olive oil or garlic infused oil, divided
- 4 cans (4.35 ounces each) sardines, drained, de-boned if required
- 1/3 cup gluten free breadcrumbs
- 6 ounces spinach leaves
- ½ teaspoon red chili flakes or to taste
- 2 tablespoons drained capers, roughly chopped
- ½ - 1 avocado, peeled, pitted, chopped
- Freshly ground pepper to taste
- Salt to taste
- 5-6 scallions, green parts only, thinly sliced
- 2 cans (14.5 ounces each) petite or regular diced tomatoes
- 12 ounces gluten free spaghetti
- Lemon wedges to serve

Method:

1. Place a large skillet over medium heat. Add 4 teaspoons oil. When the oil is

heated, add breadcrumbs and sauté until it is toasted lightly. Stir frequently.

2. Sprinkle salt and pepper and stir. Remove the breadcrumbs from the skillet and place in a bowl

3. Place the skillet back over heat. Add 2 teaspoons oil. When the oil is heated, add spinach and pepper and sauté until it wilts. Stir frequently. Remove the spinach and place in another bowl.

4. Place the skillet back over heat. Add 2 tablespoons oil. When the oil is heated, add scallions and chili flakes and sauté until it wilts.

5. Stir in the tomatoes with its juices. Increase the heat to medium high and let it cook until slightly thick. Stir occasionally.

6. Add capers and stir. Turn off the heat.

7. Cook spaghetti until al dente, following the directions on the package. Drain and add the pasta back into the cooked pot.

8. Set aside ½ cup of the cooked sauce (it can be used in some other recipe) and add rest of the sauce into the pot. Also add sardines and spinach and mix gently until well combined. Place over medium heat for a couple of minutes until hot.

9. Serve with breadcrumbs sprinkled on top. Also top with avocado and lemon wedges and serve.

Spiced Quinoa with Almonds and Feta

Serves: 6

Ingredients:

- 1 ½ tablespoons olive oil
- ¾ teaspoon turmeric
- 2.6 ounces flaked toasted almonds
- ½ cup parsley, chopped
- 2 tablespoons lemon juice or to taste
- 1 ½ teaspoons ground coriander
- 16 ounces quinoa, rinsed
- 5.3 ounces feta cheese, crumbled
- 4 cups boiling water

Method:

1. Place a large skillet over medium heat. Add oil. When the oil is heated, add turmeric and coriander powders and sauté for a few seconds until aromatic.
2. Add quinoa and stir-fry for a minute or so. You will be able to hear mild sounds of the quinoa popping.
3. Pour water and stir. Lower heat and cook until all the water has been absorbed and quinoa is tender.

4. Cool for a few minutes. Add rest of the ingredients and fluff gently and mix into it.
5. Serve either warm or cold.

Vegan Coconut Green Curry

Serves: 3

Ingredients:

- 1 teaspoon coconut oil or garlic infused oil
- 1 medium potato, peeled, cut into 1 inch cubes
- 1 cup spinach, shredded
- 1 small head broccoli, cut into florets
- 1 small courgette, chopped
- ½ inch ginger, peeled, minced
- ½ cup coconut milk
- ½ teaspoon ground cumin
- ¼ teaspoon red chili flakes
- ½ teaspoon ground turmeric
- 1 teaspoon lime juice
- A handful fresh cilantro, chopped (optional)
- A fistful cashews, chopped (optional)
- ½ cup water
- Salt to taste

Method:

1. Place a skillet over medium heat. Add oil. When the oil is heated, add ginger, turmeric and cumin and sauté for a few seconds until fragrant.

2. Add potatoes and sauté for a while. Sprinkle some water if the potatoes are getting stuck to the bottom of the pan.
3. Add broccoli and courgette and stir. Stir in coconut milk, salt and water.
4. Cover and cook until the vegetables are soft. Turn off the heat.
5. Add spinach, lime juice and chili flakes. Stir and cover for a few minutes.
6. Taste and adjust the lime, salt and chili flakes if necessary.
7. Sprinkle cilantro and cashew on top and serve.

Spicy Potato Pie

Serves: 6-8

Ingredients:

- 6 large potatoes, peeled, grated
- 1-2 red chilies, finely chopped
- 1 ½ tablespoons cooking oil
- 9 rashers bacon
- 6 eggs
- Salt to taste
- Pepper to taste
- 5 spring onions, green parts only, thinly sliced
- 3 teaspoons garlic infused oil
- 1 ½ red bell peppers, finely chopped
- 1 ½ bags baby spinach leaves, cut into thin strips
- ¼ cup rice flour
- ¼ cup tapioca flour, mixed

Method:

1. Place a skillet over medium heat. Add cooking oil and garlic infused oil. When the oils are heated, add chili and spring onions and sauté until tender.
2. Add bacon and cook for a while. Turn off heat. When cool enough to handle chop bacon into chunks.

3. Squeeze the potatoes of excess moisture. Add into a bowl. Add rest of the ingredients and mix well.
4. Transfer into a greased tart pan. Spread it evenly.
5. Bake in a preheated oven at 350° F for about 30-45 minutes.

Shepherd's Pie

Serves: 6

Ingredients:

- 2 tablespoons vegetable oil
- 4 carrots, peeled, chopped
- 2 large parsnips, peeled, chopped
- 8 cups meat stock
- 6-8 floury potatoes like King Edward or Maris Piper, peeled, chopped
- A little rice milk or lactose free milk
- 2 teaspoons fresh rosemary or thyme
- 1 swede, peeled, chopped
- 14 ounces canned chopped tomatoes
- 22 ounces cold leftover roast lamb, finely chopped
- 2-3 tablespoons lactose free butter

Method:

1. Place a heavy bottomed pan over medium heat. Add oil. When the oil is heated, add carrots, rosemary, parsnip and swede and sauté until brown.
2. Add tomatoes and stock and stir.
3. When it begins to boil, lower heat and simmer. Add lamb and simmer until the liquid in the pan is reduced to 2/3 its original quantity. The sauce would have been thicker by now.
4. Turn off the heat and pour into a heatproof casserole dish. Let it cool for a while.

5. Meanwhile, place a pot, half filled with water and a little salt over medium heat. Add potatoes and cook until potatoes are soft.
6. Drain and mash the potatoes with a potato masher. Add butter and the milk you are using and mash until creamy.
7. Layer the meat mixture with mashed potato. Spread it evenly.
8. Bake in a preheated oven at 350 °F for 40-50 minutes or until the top is golden brown.

Spanish Chicken with Paprika Potatoes

Serve: 4

Ingredients:

- 2 baking potatoes, peeled, cubed
- 1 tablespoon smoked paprika
- 3 jarred roasted peppers, finely chopped
- 5 tablespoons lactose free cream cheese
- 2-3 tablespoons lactose free butter
- 1 tablespoon olive oil
- 2 teaspoons balsamic vinegar
- 4 chicken thighs, skinless, boneless
- 2 cups mixed salad leaves
- Salt to taste
- Pepper to taste

Method:

1. Spread the potatoes on a baking sheet.
2. Add ½ tablespoon paprika, ½ tablespoon oil, 1-teaspoon vinegar, salt and pepper into a bowl and stir. Sprinkle over the potatoes and toss well.
3. Bake in a preheated oven at 390 °F for 10 minutes.
4. Add pepper, cream cheese, salt and pepper into a bowl and mix well.
5. Open up the chicken thighs and stuff the cream cheese mixture in it. Bring together the edges of the chicken and enclose the stuffing. Place the chicken

with its seam side facing down on a foil. Have one foil for each chicken thigh.

6. Add smoked paprika and butter into a small bowl. Place a little of the butter mixture on each chicken. Wrap the chicken completely in the foil.

7. Place the foil packets on top of the potatoes. Bake for another 30 minutes until the potatoes are crunchy and the chicken is cooked through.

8. Meanwhile, add remaining oil and vinegar in a small bowl and pour over the salad leaves.

9. Divide the salad into individual serving plates. Place chicken over the salad leaves.

10. Serve paprika potatoes on the side.

Stir Fry Chili Pork

Serves: 4-5

Ingredients:

- 1 ½ tablespoons gluten free soy sauce
- 1 ½ tablespoons sesame oil
- 1.3 pounds pork fillet, cut into thin slices
- 1 ½ teaspoons garlic infused oil
- 3 scallions, green part only, thinly sliced
- 20 ounces cooked rice noodles, to serve
- 3 tablespoons mirin
- 1 ½ teaspoons dried chili flakes
- 4 ½ tablespoons sunflower or vegetable oil
- 4 red chilies, halved lengthwise, do not discard stalk, deseeded
- 3 tablespoons granulated sugar

Method:

1. Add mirin, soy sauce, sesame oil and chili flakes into a bowl and stir.
2. Add pork and mix until well coated. Place in the refrigerator for 15-20 minutes.
3. Place a wok over high heat. Add 1-½ tablespoons of oil. When the oil is heated, add pork and sauté for a couple of minutes. Remove pork with a slotted spoon and set aside.
4. Add remaining oil into the wok. When the oil heats, add chilies, rice noodles

and about 1-2 tablespoons water. Sauté
for a couple of minutes.
5. Lower heat and place a lid on the wok.
   Cook for 2-3 minutes. Stir in the soy
   sauce and sugar and add the pork back
   into the wok. Stir-fry for a minute.
6. Turn off the heat. Add scallion greens
   and serve right away.

Pork Loin Roast with Herb Stuffing

Serves: 5

Ingredients:

- 2 ¾ pounds pork loin roast
- 1 cup low FODMAP chicken stock
- ½ tablespoon olive oil
- ½ cup fresh parsley, chopped
- ½ teaspoon dried oregano
- 1 ½ tablespoons pumpkin seeds
- ½ cup medium grain white rice like Arborio rice
- ¾ cup leeks, green part only
- ½ tablespoon garlic infused oil
- 1 green onion or scallion, green part only, thinly sliced
- ¼ teaspoon dried thyme
- Rock salt to taste

Method:

1. Place a saucepan over medium heat. Add olive oil and garlic infused oil. When the oil is heated, add leeks and sauté for a couple of minutes.
2. Stir in the rice and cook for a couple of minutes.
3. Add stock, a little at a time and cook until the stock is absorbed each time.

Cook until rice is done and sticky but not runny. Turn off the heat.

4. Add parsley, herbs, scallions and pumpkin seeds and mix well. Transfer into a bowl and set aside to cool.
5. Stuff this filling inside the pork roast. Tie up the roast after stuffing. Rub the outside of the pork with a little oil. Sprinkle salt liberally over it and place in a roasting pan.
6. Roast in a preheated oven at 430 °F for 30 minutes.
7. Baste the pork with the juices released. Sprinkle salt lightly.
8. Lower the temperature to 390 °F. Roast until cooked through.
9. Remove the pork from the oven and place on your cutting board.
10. When cool enough to handle, slice and serve with a vegetable side dish of your choice and cranberry sauce, preferably homemade.

One Pot Chicken and Rice

Serves: 6

Ingredients:

- 6 chicken breasts, skinless, boneless
- ½ teaspoon black pepper
- ½ teaspoon sea salt
- 2 ½ teaspoons ground cumin, divided
- 1 ½ tablespoons coconut oil
- 2 medium tomatoes, chopped
- 1 ½ teaspoons turmeric powder
- 3 cups Casa De Santa Low FODMAP vegetable stock to be made by mixing 3 teaspoons stock with 3 cups of hot water
- 1 ½ cups rice, rinsed
- 4 cups spinach, shredded
- 1 large red bell pepper, deseeded, chopped
- 1 green bell pepper, deseeded, chopped

Method:

1. Place a chicken breast on a plastic wrap. Place another wrap on the chicken. Pound with a meat mallet until it is thick evenly.
2. Repeat with the remaining chicken pieces.

3. Sprinkle salt, pepper, a little of the paprika and a little of the cumin on both sides of the chicken.
4. Place a large skillet over medium high heat. Add chicken and cook until brown on both the sides. Remove chicken with a slotted spoon and set aside.
5. Add bell peppers, ginger and tomatoes into the skillet and cook until tender.
6. Add remaining cumin and paprika. Cook for a few seconds until fragrant.
7. Add rice and sauté until rice is well coated with the mixture.
8. Add stock and stir. Add chicken back into the skillet.
9. Cover the pan with a fitting lid.
10. Lower heat and cook until most of the stock is absorbed.
11. Add spinach and cook until it wilts.
12. Sprinkle cilantro on top and serve.

Mozzarella Chicken

Serves: 2

Ingredients:

- 2 chicken breasts, skinless, boneless
- ½ tablespoons garlic infused oil
- 1 medium carrot, finely chopped
- 1 small stalk celery, finely chopped
- 7.5 ounces canned chopped tomatoes
- 1 teaspoon dried oregano
- 4.5 ounces low fat mozzarella cheese, sliced, drained on paper towels
- Cooking oil spray
- 1 ½ tablespoons tomato puree
- 1 ½ ounces green or black olives, pitted

Method:

1. Preheat a grill on high setting.
2. Sprinkle salt and pepper over the chicken.
3. Place a heatproof pan over high heat. Spray with cooking spray.
4. Add chicken and cook for 3 minutes per side or until light brown on both the sides. Remove with a slotted spoon and set aside on a plate.

5. Lower heat to low heat. Add tomatoes, tomato puree, olives and oregano and stir.
6. Cook for 4-5 minutes. Stir frequently. Pour tomato mixture over the chicken. Place mozzarella slices on top. Season with pepper.
7. Grill for a few minutes until cheese melts.

Quiche Lorraine

Serves: 6

Ingredients:

For crust:

- 1 cup rice flour
- 1 cup tapioca starch
- 1 cup millet flour
- ½ cup butter
- ½ - ¾ cup water
- 1 teaspoon salt
- 2 tablespoons apple cider vinegar

For filling:

- 7 ounces bacon, finely chopped
- 4 tablespoons Greek yogurt
- 3 ounces Gruyere cheese, grated or diced
- A pinch salt
- 4 eggs
- 1 cup lactose free milk
- 1 teaspoon nutmeg
- Pepper to taste

Method:

1. To make crust: Add flour, tapioca starch, salt and butter in a bowl. Use your fingertips and mix the ingredients until small pea size bits are formed.

2. Add vinegar and mix well.
3. Add water, a tablespoon at a time and mix well each time. Knead into a smooth and elastic dough. Add more water if the dough is not nice and smooth.
4. Place a nonstick pan over medium heat. Add bacon and cook until crisp. Turn off the heat. Set aside to cool.
5. Place dough in the refrigerator for an hour or so to chill.
6. To make filling: Add eggs, milk and Greek yogurt into a bowl and whisk well.
7. Add bacon and stir.
8. Divide the dough into 2 large tart pans or 6 smaller tart pans. Press on to the bottom as well as the sides of the pan.
9. Poke the bottom of the dough with a fork all over. Spread the filling over it.
10. Bake in a preheated oven at 350 °F for 50 minutes or until brown and cooked.
11. Let it cool for 8-10 minutes.
12. Serve hot or cold with a green salad on the side.

Maple and Sesame Chicken with Brown Rice

Serves: 8

Ingredients:

- 8 teaspoons maple syrup
- 2 pounds chicken thighs, skinless, boneless
- ½ teaspoon salt
- 2 teaspoons sesame seeds
- 2 teaspoons black sesame seeds
- ¼ cup fresh cilantro, chopped
- 8 teaspoons gluten free soy sauce
- 10 ounces brown rice
- 1 teaspoon vegetable oil
- 2 teaspoons pumpkin seeds, chopped

To serve:

- 2 tablespoons sesame oil
- 4 heads Bok Choy, halved
- 2 tablespoons rapeseed oil

Method:

1. Add maple syrup and soy sauce into a bowl. Add chicken and turn the chicken until well coated.

2. Transfer into a heavy bottomed saucepan.
3. Place the saucepan over medium heat. Cook until chicken is tender and the sauce is well glazed on the chicken.
4. Meanwhile, add rice, salt and 21 ounces water into a pan. Place the pan over medium heat.
5. When it begins to boil, lower heat and cover with a lid. Cook until tender. When done, using a fork, fluff the rice.
6. Add vegetable oil, cilantro and sesame seeds
7. Place another pan over medium heat. Add sesame oil and rapeseed oil. When the pan is heated, add Bok Choy and cook until it wilts.
8. Serve chicken over rice with Bok Choy on the side.

Chapter Six: Vegetarian Recipes

Parsnip Soup with Carrot, Coconut and Ginger

Serves: 6

Ingredients:

- 6 parsnips, peeled, chopped into small chunks
- 12 carrots, peeled, chopped into small chunks
- 6 cups FODMAP friendly vegetable stock
- 1 ½ tablespoons apple cider vinegar
- 1 ½ tablespoons paprika
- Pepper to taste
- Salt to taste
- 2 inches piece ginger, peeled, chopped
- 6 tablespoons coconut milk
- ¾ teaspoon turmeric powder
- Salt to taste
- Freshly cracked pepper to taste

Method:

1. Add carrots, parsnips and ginger into a soup pot.
2. Place the soup pot over medium heat. When the water begins to boil, add

turmeric, salt, paprika and pepper and stir.

3. Lower heat and cook until vegetables are tender.

4. Cool for a while. Transfer into a blender and blend until smooth.

5. Add coconut milk and vinegar and blend until smooth.

6. Ladle into soup bowls. Drizzle some extra coconut milk if desired. Sprinkle pumpkin seeds on top and serve.

Carrot and Fennel Soup

Serves: 6

Ingredients:

- 3 large carrots, cut into small pieces
- 2/3 pound sweet potato or parsnip, cut into small pieces
- 1.1 pound potato, cut into small pieces
- ¾ cup leeks, green part only, thinly sliced
- 1 ½ tablespoons olive oil
- 1 ½ tablespoons garlic infused oil
- 4 ½ cups low FODMAP vegetable stock
- 3 teaspoons fennel seeds
- ¾ cup low FODMAP milk
- 12 slices low FODMAP bread
- 1 ½ tablespoons dairy free spread or olive oil
- A large handful fresh cilantro, chopped, divided + extra to garnish
- Salt to taste
- Pepper to taste

Method:

1. Add both the oils in a saucepan. Place the saucepan over low heat. Add leeks and sauté for a couple of minutes. Stir occasionally.

2. Add vegetables and stir. Cook for 5 minutes. Stir once during these 5 minutes.
3. Add stock. Raise the heat to medium high heat and bring to the boil. Cover with lid and lower the heat. Simmer until vegetables are soft.
4. Meanwhile, Place a frying pan over medium heat. Add dairy free spread or olive oil. When the oil heats, add fennel seeds. Stir constantly for a minute. Add cilantro and stir.
5. After a minute, turn off the heat. Transfer into the simmering soup.
6. Add cilantro and simmer for a minute. Turn off the heat. Cool for a while. Blend in a blender until smooth. Pour soup back into the saucepan. Add milk, salt and pepper and place over low heat.
7. Ladles into soup bowls. Sprinkle some more cilantro and serve with bread.

Rolling Fresh Spring Rolls

Serves: 20-25

Ingredients:

- 20 spring roll wrappers
- 1 medium zucchini or cucumber, cut into matchsticks
- 1 ½ cups purple green beans or purple cabbage, thinly sliced
- 3 cups romaine lettuce leaves or kale or spinach, shredded
- 1 ½ bunches cilantro, chopped
- 2 bell peppers, thinly sliced
- 3 avocadoes, peeled, pitted, thinly sliced
- 2 scallions, chopped
- Sauce of your choice

Method:

1. Moisten your countertop. Add very warm water into a large bowl. Hydrate one spring roll wrapper at a time until malleable.
2. Place the rest of the ingredients along the center of the wrap, in a rectangular shape. Roll the spring roll like the way you roll a burrito.

Easy **One-Pan Ratatouille**

Serves: 4

Ingredients:

- 2 tablespoons olive oil
- 1 small zucchini
- 3 ounces thin green beans (haricot verts)
- ½ teaspoon dried herbs of your choice
- 3 tablespoons olives, chopped
- A handful fresh basil, chopped
- ½ pound eggplant, chopped
- 1 medium red bell pepper, chopped
- Salt to taste
- Pepper to taste
- 1 ¼ cups canned diced tomatoes, unsalted
- Red chili flakes to taste
- 2 ounces feta cheese, crumbled

Method:

1. Place a skillet over medium high heat. Add eggplant. Sprinkle salt and pepper and sauté until light brown.
2. Remove the eggplant from the pan and place in a bowl. Scrape the bottom of the pan by adding a little water or red wine.
3. Add about 2 teaspoons oil. Add bell pepper and zucchini and sauté on medium high heat. Sprinkle salt and

pepper. Cook until light brown. Transfer into the bowl of eggplant.

4. Add a little water and scrape the bottom of the pan to remove any browned bits.
5. Add a little oil and green beans and cook until light brown. Add tomatoes and cook until it begins to simmer.
6. Add the eggplant, bell pepper and zucchini back into the pan. Also, add herbs and chili flakes and mix well.
7. Lower heat and cover with a lid. Cook until soft and the gravy is thickened. Add more water if required. Add salt and pepper. Add olives and mix well.
8. Serve over gluten free pasta or polenta or quinoa or any other favorite dish of yours that can pair well with it.
9. Garnish with feta and basil and serve.

Pumpkin and Carrot Risotto

Serves: 6

Ingredients:

<u>For roast vegetables:</u>

- 1 pound Japanese pumpkin or Kabocha squash or Buttercup squash, cut into 1.5 cm pieces
- 2 tablespoons olive oil
- 1 pound carrots, cut into 1.5 cm pieces
- Salt to taste
- Pepper to taste

<u>For risotto:</u>

- 3 cups medium grain white rice
- 2 tablespoons garlic infused oil
- 8 cups low FODMAP vegetable stock
- 5 tablespoons lemon juice
- 1/3 cup fresh cilantro, chopped
- 1 cup leeks, green parts only, chopped
- 2 tablespoons dairy free spread or olive oil or butter
- 4 teaspoons lemon zest, grated
- 8 cups spinach, shredded
- 3.5 ounces parmesan cheese or soy based vegan cheese, grated (optional)

Method:

1. Place pumpkin and carrots in a baking dish. Drizzle oil over it. Sprinkle salt and pepper and toss well.
2. Bake in a preheated oven at 390 °F for 20-25 minutes or until brown and cooked.
3. Stir the contents every 10 minutes.
4. Meanwhile, make risotto as follows: Place a saucepan over medium heat. Add dairy free spread and garlic infused oil. When the oil is heated, add rice and cook until it is well coated with the oil.
5. Add stock, a little at a time and cook until dry each time. Keep doing this until the rice cooks.
6. Add spinach, lemon zest, lemon juice, salt and pepper and mix well.
7. Add the roasted vegetables, cilantro and cheese and mix until well combined.
8. Spoon into bowls and serve.

Crunchy Roasted Potatoes

Serves: 4-6

Ingredients:

- 2.4 pounds potatoes, cubed (do not peel)
- ½ teaspoon cumin
- Pepper to taste
- Salt to taste
- 2 teaspoons ground paprika
- A pinch chili powder or to taste
- Olive oil, as required

Method:

1. Add potatoes into a bowl. Toss well oil and all the spices.
2. Spread on a baking sheet that is lined with parchment paper.
3. Bake in a preheated oven at 440 °F for 20-25 minutes or until brown and cooked.
4. Stir the contents every 12-15 minutes.
5. Serve hot.

Mushroom Polenta with Goat's Cheese

Serves: 4

Ingredients:

- 7 ounces canned mushrooms, drained, rinsed
- 10.5 ounces oyster mushrooms, scrubbed, chopped into small pieces
- 2 tablespoons truffle infused olive oil
- 4 tablespoons olive oil
- 7 ounces polenta
- 1 teaspoon rosemary
- 2 ounces goat's cheese, crumbled
- 1 low FODMAP stock cube
- 2 cubes butter
- 1.5 ounces parmesan cheese

Method:

1. Dry the canned mushrooms with paper towels.
2. Place a pan over medium heat. Add olive oil. When the oil is heated, add the mushrooms and sauté for 4-5 minutes.
3. Add truffle infused oil, pepper and salt and stir. Remove from heat and cover with a lid.
4. Meanwhile, add 4 cups water into a saucepan. Place the saucepan over medium heat. Add stock cubes and stir.

5. When it begins to boil, add polenta stirring constantly with a wooden spoon.
6. Lower heat and keep stirring until it reaches the consistency you desire. Remove from heat.
7. Add Parmesan cheese, butter and rosemary and mix until well combined.
8. Serve in individual serving plates. Top with mushroom mixture and goat's cheese.
9. Serve right away.

Pita Pizza with Grilled Vegetables

Serves: 6

Ingredients:

- 6 gluten free pitas
- 6 tomatoes, cut into thin, round slices
- 2 medium eggplants, cut into slices cross wise and then into strips (optional)
- 3 sweet red bell peppers, cut into thin slices
- 15 ounces tomato passata
- Pepper to taste
- Salt to taste
- Grated cheese, to taste (low FODMAP friendly)

Method:

1. Use eggplant only if you can tolerate it.
2. Cut each of the pizzas into 2 by using scissors along the edges. So you end up in 12 pizza bases.
3. Smear tomato passata over the pita halves.
4. Place tomatoes, bell peppers and eggplant in a grill pan. Brush with olive oil.
5. Grill on a preheated trill.
6. Spread the vegetables on the pita bases. Sprinkle salt and pepper on top.

7. Sprinkle cheese.
8. Bake in a preheated oven at 375 °F for 15 minutes.
9. Serve with a salad of your choice that can help your gut.

Quinoa Bowl with Sweet Potato and Tahini Dressing

Serves: 4

Ingredients:

For quinoa bowl:

- 8.5 ounces quinoa
- 2 medium cucumbers, sliced
- 1 medium sweet potato, peeled, cubed
- 14 ounces cherry tomatoes, halved
- 1 low FODMAP stock cube
- A handful black olives, sliced
- ½ avocado, peeled, pitted, chopped
- A handful fresh parsley, chopped

For dressing:

- 4 tablespoons tahini
- Lemon juice to taste
- 2 tablespoons water
- Pepper to taste
- Salt to taste

Method:

1. Spread the sweet potato cubes on a baking sheet. Drizzle oil over it.
2. Bake in a preheated oven at 390 °F for 15 -20 minutes or until crisp.

3. Cook quinoa following the directions on the package. Add stock cube while cooking the quinoa.
4. To make dressing: Add all the ingredients of dressing into a bowl and whisk well.
5. To assemble: Take 4 bowls. Divide the quinoa among the bowls. Layer with sweet potato followed by cucumber, olives, tomatoes and avocado.
6. Drizzle the dressing over the bowls. Sprinkle parsley on top and serve.

Pasta Muhammara

Serves: 4

Ingredients:

- 11 ounces gluten free pasta
- A handful fresh basil, chopped
- 2-3 cups vegetables of your choice
- 4 tablespoons nutritional yeast or grated cheese, to taste

For Muhammara:

- 6 roasted red peppers
- 3 tablespoons pomegranate syrup
- 2 teaspoons ground cumin
- Salt to taste
- Pepper to taste
- 2 tablespoons olive oil
- A handful walnuts
- 6 tablespoons oat flour
- ¼ teaspoon cayenne pepper
- Lemon juice to taste

Method:

1. To make muhammara: Add all the ingredients of muhammara into the food processor bowl. Pulse until smooth and well combined.
2. If muhammara is watery, add some more oats and blend again. If it is very

thick, add some more olive oil or lemon juice and blend again.

3. To make pasta: Cook pasta following the directions on the package. Drain and set aside.

4. Place a skillet over medium low heat. Spray with cooking spray. Add the vegetables that you are using and cook until done.

5. Take 4 bowls and spoon pasta among them. Spoon muhammara sauce over the pasta.

6. Sprinkle basil and nutritional yeast and serve.

Tempeh Goreng

Serves: 4-6

Ingredients:

- 1.1 pound tempeh, cut into slices of ½ cm thickness
- 3-4 teaspoons sambal
- 2 teaspoons fresh ginger, grated
- 1/8 teaspoon salt or to taste
- 14 ounces sunflower oil
- 8 tablespoons ketjap (sweet soy sauce)
- 2 teaspoons sugar

Method:

1. Place a heatproof pan over medium heat. Add oil. When the oil is heated, add tempeh in batches and fry until brown and crisp. Remove with a slotted spoon and place on a plate that is lined with paper towels.
2. Place another pan over medium heat. Add a little of the leftover oil. Add ginger, sugar, sambal, ketjap and salt and stir for 5-6 seconds.
3. Add tempeh and sauté for a while. Stir frequently. In a while, ketjap will form a glaze around the tempeh.

4. Serve right away. Tastes great with rice or vegetables.

Vegan Tostadas with Tofu

Serves: 4

Ingredients:

- 12-15 corn tortillas
- 4 tomatoes, chopped
- 14 ounces tofu, drained, crumbled
- 2 bell peppers, topped
- 2 teaspoons ground cumin
- ½ teaspoon turmeric powder
- ½ teaspoon ground cinnamon
- 2 teaspoons smoked paprika
- ½ teaspoon chili powder
- 1 avocado, peeled, pitted, chopped
- 4 tablespoons nutritional yeast or grated cheese (optional)
- A handful fresh cilantro, chopped
- Lactose free cream cheese to serve
- Salt to taste
- Pepper to taste
- Lemon juice to taste
- 7 ounces canned mushrooms

Method:

1. Add bell pepper and tomatoes into a baking dish. Drizzle some oil over it. Toss well.
2. Bake in a preheated oven at 350 °F for 15 minutes or until slightly soft. Add

mushroom and bake for another 10-15 minutes.

3. Add tofu and spices and toss well. Bake for another 10 minutes. Stir a couple of times while it is baking.

4. Place the tortillas on a baking sheet. Brush with a little oil. Bake for 5 minutes. Flip sides and bake for 2-3 minutes.

5. Add avocado into a bowl. Drizzle lemon juice over it and toss well.

6. Place tortillas on individual serving plates. Spread tofu mushroom mixture over the tortillas.

7. Sprinkle avocado and cilantro and nutritional yeast if using.

8. Serve right away.

Chapter Seven: Dessert Recipes

Banana Ice Cream

Serves: 10-12

Ingredients:

- 2 cans (14 ounces each) light coconut milk
- 2 teaspoons vanilla bean paste or extract
- 4 bananas, peeled, sliced
- ½ cup dark chocolate chips (optional)

Method:

1. Pour 1½ cans of coconut milk into ice an ice cube tray. Freeze until firm. Chill the remaining coconut milk.
2. Place bananas on a freezer safe tray and freeze until firm.
3. Add frozen bananas, coconut milk ice cubes, vanilla and coconut milk into a blender. Pulse until creamy.
4. Scoop into bowls. Sprinkle chocolate chips on top and serve.

Chocolate Peanut Butter Chia Pudding

Serves: 6-8 (1/3 cup each)

Ingredients:

- ½ cup chia seeds
- 2 tablespoons natural creamy peanut butter
- 2 tablespoons pure maple syrup
- 2 tablespoons cocoa powder, unsweetened
- 2 cups canned light coconut milk

Method:

1. Add all the ingredients into a jar with a lid or use a mason's jar.
2. Close the lid and shake the jar vigorously.
3. Uncover and stir with a spoon. Cover and shake the jar vigorously once more.
4. Chill for 4-6 hours.
5. Serve as it is or serve with fruits.

Frosted Biscotti

Serves:

Ingredients:

- 3 tablespoons butter, at room temperature
- 2 eggs
- 3 teaspoons baking powder
- 3 teaspoons vegetable oil
- 2 teaspoons almond extract
- 2 teaspoons vanilla extract
- 1 cup sugar
- 3 cups gluten free all-purpose flour blend
- 2/3 cup lactose free milk

For icing:

- 1 ½ -2 cups confectioner's sugar
- 1 teaspoon vanilla extract
- 4 tablespoons butter, at room temperature
- 2-3 teaspoons lactose free milk

Method:

1. Add butter and sugar into a mixing bowl. Beat with an electric mixer until smooth and creamy.
2. Add eggs, one at a time and beat well each time.

3. Mix together flour and baking powder and add into the bowl. Mix until well combined.
4. Add oil, vanilla and almond extracts and mix well.
5. Line a large baking sheet with parchment paper. You 2 baking sheets if required.
6. Drop large spoonful of batter on the prepared baking sheet. Leave a gap between 2 cookies.
7. Bake in a preheated oven at 350° F for about 20 minutes or until the edges are light brown.
8. Remove from the oven and let it cool for 5-8 minutes on the baking sheet. Loosen the cookies with a metal spatula. Cool completely.
9. Meanwhile, make the icing as follows: Add 1 cup confectioner's sugar, vanilla, butter and milk into a bowl and whisk well. Add remaining sugar and beat until creamy.
10. Spread a thin layer of the icing over the biscotti. Cut if desired and serve.
11. Store in an airtight container.

Chocolate Coconut Cookies

Serves:

Ingredients:

- 2 sticks butter, at room temperature
- 2 eggs
- 1 cup 60% cacao chocolate chips, melted, slightly cooled
- 1 cup whole grain brown rice flour
- ½ cup chopped, shredded sweetened coconut
- 2/3 cup granulated sugar
- 2 teaspoons vanilla extract
- 2 cups gluten free flour blend
- 2 teaspoons baking soda

Method:

1. Add butter and sugar into a mixing bowl. Beat with an electric mixer until smooth and creamy.
2. Add eggs, one at a time and beat well each time. Add chocolate and fold gently.
3. Mix together flour and baking powder and add into the bowl. Mix until well combined.
4. Add vanilla and mix well. Add coconut and mix to form dough.

5. Line a large baking sheet with parchment paper. You 2 baking sheets if required. Set aside.
6. Roll the dough into a cylindrical shape of about 2-½ inches diameter.
7. Wrap the dough with parchment paper and chill for 2-3 hours or until hard.
8. Remove the dough and place on your cutting board. Cut into 1/3 inch thick slices.
9. Place on the prepared baking sheet.
10. Bake in a preheated oven at 350° F for about 20 minutes or until the edges are light brown.
11. Remove from the oven and let it cool for 5-8 minutes on the baking sheet. Loosen the cookies with a metal spatula. Cool completely.
12. Store in an airtight container.

Pumpkin Crumb Cake

Serves: 6-8

Ingredients:

<u>For toppings:</u>

- ¼ cup granulated sugar
- ¼ cup pecans, chopped
- 1/3 cup gluten free flour blend
- 6 tablespoons melted butter or coconut oil

<u>For filling:</u>

- 3 tablespoons brown sugar
- ½ -1 teaspoon cocoa powder, unsweetened
- ½ teaspoon cinnamon

<u>For cake:</u>

- 3 tablespoons vegetable oil
- ½ cup sugar
- ½ teaspoon salt
- ¾ teaspoon gluten free flour blend
- 1 large egg
- ½ cup pumpkin puree
- ¼ teaspoon salt
- ½ teaspoon pumpkin pie spice

Method:

1. Grease a small baking pan with a little oil.
2. Add all the topping ingredients into a bowl and mix until crumbly.
3. Add all filling ingredients into a bowl. Mix well.
4. To make the cake: Add oil, egg, pumpkin pie spice, pumpkin puree and sugar into a bowl and whisk with an electric mixer until well combined.
5. Add baking powder, salt and flour and whisk until lightly combined.
6. Spoon half the batter into the prepared pan. Spread filling over it. Spread remaining batter over the filling.
7. Take a blunt knife and swirl the mixture lightly.
8. Sprinkle topping mixture all over the top.
9. Bake in a preheated oven at 350 °F for 35-40 minutes.

Chocolate Peanut Butter Bits

Serves: 10-12 (2 balls per serving)

Ingredients:

- ½ cup semi-sweet chocolate chips
- 2/3 cup all natural peanut butter
- 2 teaspoons vanilla paste or extract
- ½ cup shredded coconut, unsweetened
- ½ cup oat bran
- 1 cup rolled oats
- ½ cup walnuts, chopped
- 2 tablespoons maple syrup

Method:

1. Add all the ingredients into the food processor bowl and pulse until well combined.
2. If the mixture is too dry (you are not able to form balls) add a little more maple syrup. If the mixture is too runny, add a little more oat bran.
3. Divide the mixture into 20-25 portions and shape into balls.

Creamy Coconut Milk Quinoa Pudding

Serves:

Ingredients:

- 1 ½ cups uncooked quinoa, drained, rinsed
- 4 tablespoons pure maple syrup
- A handful fresh blueberries
- 2 tablespoons whipped cream
- 2 cans (14 ounces each) light coconut milk
- 2 teaspoons vanilla extract or vanilla bean paste
- Walnuts or almonds, chopped (optional)

Method:

1. Add coconut milk and quinoa into a saucepan. Place the saucepan over high heat. When it begins to boil, lower heat and add maple syrup and vanilla extract.
2. Cook until tender and the consistency is of pudding.
3. Turn off the heat. Refrigerate until it cools slightly.
4. Spoon into dessert bowls. Sprinkle blueberries on top and decorate with a little bit of cream. Sprinkle chopped almonds or walnuts, if using and serve.

Coconut Milk Soft Serve "Ice Cream"

Serves: 3 cups

- Frozen unsweetened coconut milk
- 2 tablespoons packed brown sugar
- ½ cup mini chocolate chips
- A little coconut milk or water
- 2 teaspoons vanilla extract

Method:

1. To make frozen coconut milk, pour coconut milk into ice cube trays and freeze until firm.
2. Remove the cubes and add into a blender. Also, add brown sugar and vanilla. Add a little coconut milk if necessary. Blend until combine.
3. Scoop into bowls. Top with mini chocolate chips on top and serve.

Double Chocolate Flourless Cookies with Salted Peanuts

Serves:

- ½ cup cocoa powder
- 2 teaspoons baking soda
- 1 cup peanut butter
- 2/3 cup semi-sweet chocolate chips
- 2/3 cup firmly packed brown sugar
- 2 extra-large eggs
- 2 teaspoons vanilla
- 2/3 cup salted peanuts, roughly chopped

Method:

1. Line 3-4 baking sheets with parchment paper. Set aside.
2. Add brown sugar, cocoa and baking soda into a bowl and stir.
3. Add eggs, peanut butter and vanilla into a bowl and whisk until well combined. If the mixture is too dry, add 1-2 teaspoons oil and whisk.
4. Add chocolate chips and peanuts and fold gently.
5. Make balls of about 1-½ inches diameter and place on the baking sheet. Leave a gap between 2 cookies. Flatten slightly if desired.

6. Bake in a preheated oven at 350 °F for 8 minutes.

Two Bite Frosted Brownies

Serves: 20-25

Ingredients:

- 1 cup gluten free flour
- 2 tablespoons granulated sugar
- 1 cup semi-sweet or bitter sweet chocolate chips
- 2 teaspoons vanilla
- 1 teaspoon baking soda
- 8 tablespoons butter
- 4 eggs, beaten

For frosting:

- 8 tablespoons butter, at room temperature
- 1 ½ cups confectioner's sugar
- 2 teaspoons vanilla extract
- 4 teaspoons lactose free milk

Method:

1. Line 2 mini muffin tins of 12 count each with paper liners.
2. Add gluten free flour, sugar and baking soda into a bowl and stir.
3. Add butter and chocolate chips into a microwave safe bowl. Microwave on High for 1 minute after which in

increments of 15 seconds until melted. Whisk at each increment.

4. Pour into the bowl of flour mixture.
5. Add eggs and vanilla and beat until smooth and creamy.
6. Pour into the muffin molds. Do not fill more than ¾ the cup.
7. Bake in a preheated oven at 350 °F for 12 minutes or a toothpick, when inserted in the center, should come out clean.
8. Meanwhile, add butter and vanilla into a bowl and beat until smooth. Add confectioner's sugar and milk and beat until the desired consistency is achieved.
9. When the brownies are cooled completely, spread the frosting on top. Sprinkle sprinkles on top if desired and serve.

Frozen Banana Pops

Serves: 8

Ingredients:

- 4 bananas, peeled, halved
- 2/3 cu vanilla Greek yogurt
- 2/3 cup nuts of your choice, chopped
- 8 lollipop sticks
- 2 tablespoons all-natural peanut butter
- 2/3 cup mini chocolate chips

Method:

1. Insert the lollipop sticks in each of the banana halves.
2. Add yogurt and peanut butter in a bowl and whisk well.
3. Add nuts and chocolate chips in a tray that is lined with parchment paper.
4. Dip the bananas in the yogurt mixture.
5. Dredge in the nut mixture.
6. Place the entire tray with the bananas in the freezer.

Chocolate Chip Cheesecake in a Mug

Serves: 2

Ingredients:

- 8 ounces lactose free cream cheese
- 4 tablespoons confectioner's sugar
- ½ teaspoon vanilla extract
- 3-4 tablespoons low FODMAP cookie crumbs
- 4 tablespoons sour cream or lactose free if you cannot tolerate it
- 2 large eggs
- 2 tablespoons semi-sweet chocolate morsels

Method:

1. Spray 2 microwave safe coffee mugs with a little cooking spray.
2. Add cream cheese, confectioner's sugar, sour cream, vanilla and eggs into a bowl and whisk until smooth.
3. Add semi-sweet chocolate morsels and fold gently. Divide into the 2 prepared mugs.
4. Microwave on High for 2 minutes and 40 seconds or until the cakes are done.
5. Garnish with cookie crumbs and serve.

Chapter Eight: Dips

Arugula Feta Dip

Each serving is of ¼ cup

Ingredients:

- 8 cups baby arugula
- 4 tablespoons fresh lemon juice
- 28 ounces feta cheese
- 2-4 tablespoons garlic infused olive oil

Method:

1. Add all the ingredients into a blender and blend until smooth.
2. Transfer into a bowl and serve.

FODMAP Friendly Hummus

Each serving is of ¼ cup

Ingredients:

- 2 cans (14.5 ounces each) chickpeas, drained, rinsed
- 2 teaspoons ground cumin
- Water, as required
- 4 tablespoons lime juice
- 2 tablespoons garlic infused olive oil

Method:

1. Add all the ingredients into a blender and blend until smooth.
2. Transfer into a bowl and serve.

Berry Chia Jam

Makes: 2/3 cup

Ingredients:

- ½ cup strawberries, chopped
- 2 cups frozen wild blueberries
- 2 tablespoons chia seeds
- 3 tablespoons maple syrup
- 1 teaspoon vanilla extract

Method:

1. Add berries and maple syrup into a pan. Place the pan over medium heat.
2. In a while, the berries will begin to release its juices. Mash the berries with a potato masher.
3. Simmer until slightly thick. Add chia seeds and cook for a couple of minutes.
4. Turn off the heat. Let it cool for a while.
5. Transfer into a glass jar. Fasten the lid. Refrigerate until use.
6. It can store for 1 week in the refrigerator.

Cinnamon Raisin Farmer Cheese

Serves: 4

Ingredients:

- ½ pound farmer cheese
- 4 tablespoons maple syrup
- 2 teaspoons ground cinnamon
- 3 tablespoons golden raisins

Method:

1. Add all the ingredients into a bowl and chill.
2. Serve with FODMAP friendly crackers or gluten free bread or baby carrots.

Cranberry Nut Butter

Serves:

Ingredients:

- 1 ½ cups roasted peanuts
- ¼ cup almonds
- ½ cup walnuts
- ¼ cup dried cranberries

Method:

1. Add all the ingredients into a blender and blend until smooth.

Simple Homemade Grainy Mustard

Serves:

Ingredients:

- 2 tablespoons yellow mustard seeds
- 6 tablespoons white wine vinegar or any other vinegar of your choice
- ½ teaspoon salt
- 2 tablespoons brown mustard seeds
- ¾ teaspoon sugar
- Water, if required, a little

Method:

1. Add both the mustard seeds in a glass bowl. Pour vinegar over it. Cover the bowl with cling wrap and let it sit at room temperature for 8-9 hours.
2. Add 2/3 of the mustard mixture into a blender. Also, add salt and sugar. Pulse until smooth and well combined. Transfer into a bowl.
3. Add remaining mustard mixture and fold gently. Transfer into a glass jar. Close the lid and refrigerate until use. It can last 2-3 days.

Sweet Strawberry Refrigerator Jam

Serves:

Ingredients:

- 4 cups strawberries, chopped, rinsed, trimmed
- 2-3 tablespoons table sugar
- 2 tablespoons fresh lemon juice

Method:

1. Add all the ingredients into small saucepan. Place a saucepan over medium heat.
2. Let it boil. Stir frequently. Mash it simultaneously as it cooks, with the back of a spoon.
3. Lower heat and let it simmer for a while until thicker. Turn off heat.
4. Cool for a while. Spoon into a glass jar with a fitting lid. Place in the refrigerator. It can last for a week.

Quick and Easy Cranberry Orange Relish

Serves:

Ingredients:

- 2 bags (8 ounces each) fresh cranberries, rinsed
- ½ cup sugar
- 2 seedless oranges, peeled, separated into segments, cut into pieces, deseeded

Method:

1. Add all the ingredients into a food processor bowl and pulse until well combined

2. Transfer into a bowl. Cover and chill for 7-8 hours.

Sweet & Spicy BBQ Wing

Serves:

Ingredients:

- 3 pounds package cut chicken wings
- 1 tablespoon brown sugar
- 1 cup gluten free panko bread crumbs
- 4 tablespoons BBQ spice blend
- ¼ teaspoon salt or to taste

To serve:

- Red pepper strips
- Carrot strips

Method:

1. Line 2 baking sheets with parchment paper.
2. Add BBQ spice blend, salt and brown sugar into a bowl and mix well.
3. Transfer into a zip lock bag. Add breadcrumbs. Seal the bag and shake until well combined.
4. Add wings into the bag and shake until well coated. Transfer on to a baking sheet.
5. Bake in a preheated oven at 450 °F for 30 minutes. Turn sides half way through cooking.

Conclusion

I want to thank you once again for choosing this book. The book was written with the intent to provide you with low FODMAP recipes. The recipes mentioned in this book are easy to cook and the ingredients are easily available in your local farmer's market.

I hope the recipes help you combat your leaky gut condition.

Thank you!

Chris Power

For more information on the Leaky Gut Diet please refer to my other book "Leaky Gut Diet - The Low FODMAP Diet made easy." This book goes into a lot more detail about the syndrome and provides some detailed information on foods to include in your diet and those to avoid.

81298329R00091

Made in the USA
Middletown, DE
22 July 2018